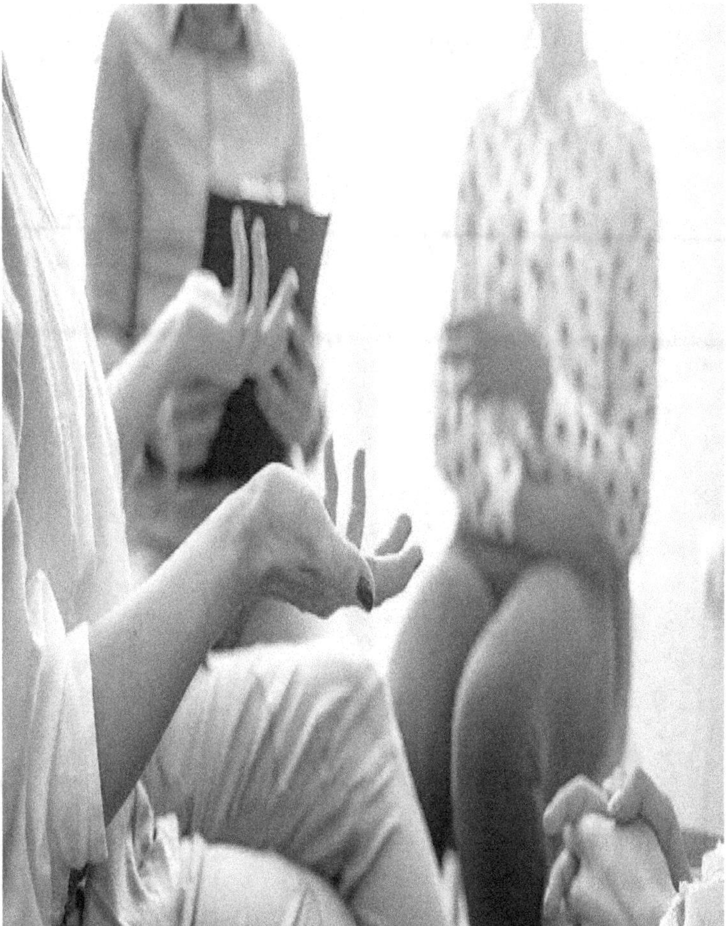

HOW NOT TO DIE

OUTLIVE CANCER

BY

ANNANTRAM A. DIVINE

COPYRIGHT

DEDICATION

Dedicated to all those who have been affected by cancer.

To those who have lost loved ones, to those who have fought and overcome, and to those who continue to battle this disease every day - this book is for you. Your strength, resilience, and courage inspire us all. We honor your journeys and remain committed to finding better treatments and a cure for cancer.

TABLE OF CONTENTS

INTRODUCTION

Cancer is one of the most feared diseases in the world. It is estimated that in 2020 alone, there were 19.3 million new cases of cancer worldwide, and 10 million cancer-related deaths. A cancer diagnosis can be overwhelming and life-changing, and the journey through treatment and recovery can be long and challenging. However, with the right information, resources, and support, it is possible to live a full and meaningful life with cancer.

This book is a practical guide to living with cancer. It is designed to help people who have been diagnosed with cancer, as well as their loved ones, navigate the complexities of cancer treatment and recovery. Whether you are newly diagnosed, in the middle of treatment, or in remission, this book offers advice, support, and encouragement for every step of the journey.

Part One of the book provides an overview of cancer, including its causes, types, and stages.

It also covers the various treatment options available, such as surgery, radiation therapy, chemotherapy, and immunotherapy. The goal of this section is to help readers understand their diagnosis and treatment options so that they can make informed decisions about their care.

Part Two of the book is focused on coping with cancer. It covers a range of topics, from managing the emotional impact of cancer to dealing with physical symptoms and side effects of treatment. Readers will also learn about the importance of self-care, such as eating a healthy diet, exercising, and getting enough sleep, as well as complementary therapies like meditation and acupuncture.

Part Three of the book is about building a support network. Cancer can be isolating, and having a network of friends, family, and healthcare professionals can make all the difference. This section offers practical advice on how to communicate effectively with loved ones and medical professionals, how to find a support group, and how to advocate for yourself throughout your cancer journey.

Part Four of the book is focused on living with uncertainty. Cancer is an unpredictable disease, and living with uncertainty can be challenging. This section offers tips on how to stay present in the moment, find joy and meaning in life despite the challenges of cancer, and maintain hope and resilience in the face of uncertainty.

Finally, Part Five of the book is about planning for the future. This section covers topics such as advance care planning, financial planning, and end-of-life care. While it can be difficult to think about these issues, planning ahead can bring a sense of peace and security and ensure that your wishes are respected.

Throughout the book, readers will find personal stories from cancer survivors, caregivers, and healthcare professionals, as well as practical advice and resources to help them navigate their cancer journey. By the end of the book, readers will have a comprehensive understanding of how to live with cancer and how to take control of their cancer journey.

The goal of this book is to empower readers to live their best life with cancer. Whether you are newly diagnosed, in the middle of treatment, or in remission, this book is here to help you navigate the challenges of cancer and find hope, resilience, and meaning in life. It is not a substitute for medical advice, but rather a supplement to it, providing readers with the information and resources they need to make informed decisions about their care and to live well with cancer.

Living with cancer is not easy, but it is possible. With the right support, resources, and mindset, you can live a full and meaningful life, even in the face of this challenging disease. This book is here to help you do just that.

Part one.

Chapter one: AN OVERVIEW OF CANCER

What is cancer:
Cancer is a disease characterized by the abnormal and uncontrolled growth of cells in the body. It occurs when the normal mechanisms that control cell growth and division become disrupted, causing cells to divide and multiply rapidly and form a mass of abnormal cells known as a tumor. Cancer can occur in any part of the body and can spread to other parts through the bloodstream or lymphatic system. There are many different types of cancer, each with its own unique characteristics and treatment options. Cancer is a complex and multifaceted disease that can have a significant impact on a person's health and well-being, as well as their family and loved ones. The treatment of cancer can involve a range of approaches, including surgery,

radiation therapy, chemotherapy, and targeted therapy, among others. With early detection and appropriate treatment, many cancers can be successfully treated, and individuals can go on to lead long and healthy lives.

Cancer is a complex disease that involves the uncontrolled growth of abnormal cells in the body. Normally, the body's cells grow and divide in a controlled manner, as new cells replace old or damaged ones. However, when this process goes awry, cells can grow and divide uncontrollably, forming a mass of abnormal cells known as a tumor.

Tumors can be either benign or malignant. Benign tumors are noncancerous and typically grow slowly, remaining confined to a particular area of the body. They do not invade nearby tissues or spread to other parts of the body. In contrast, malignant tumors are cancerous and can grow rapidly, invade nearby tissues, and spread to other parts of the body through the bloodstream or lymphatic system. The process of cancer spreading to other parts of the body is called metastasis.

There are many different types of cancer, each
with its own unique characteristics and
treatment options. Some of the most common
types of cancer include breast cancer, lung
cancer, prostate cancer, and colorectal cancer.
Each type of cancer has its own risk factors,
signs, and symptoms, as well as specific
methods for diagnosis and treatment.

Cancer can have a significant impact on a
person's health and well-being, as well as their
family and loved ones. The treatment of cancer
can involve a range of approaches, including
surgery, radiation therapy, chemotherapy,
targeted therapy, immunotherapy, and
hormone therapy, among others. The
appropriate treatment for cancer depends on
several factors, including the type of cancer, the
stage of the cancer, and the person's overall
health.

Early detection and treatment of cancer are
critical for improving outcomes and increasing
the chances of survival. This is why it is
important for individuals to be aware of the risk

factors associated with cancer and to undergo regular cancer screenings as recommended by their healthcare providers. Additionally, making healthy lifestyle choices, such as eating a balanced diet, getting regular exercise, and avoiding tobacco and excessive alcohol consumption, can help reduce the risk of developing certain types of cancer.

Going Broader on Tumor

In cancer, tumors are a mass of abnormal cells that grow and divide uncontrollably. These cells can form solid tumors or liquid tumors in the blood or lymphatic system.

Solid tumors are formed when abnormal cells divide and grow uncontrollably and form a mass or lump that can be felt or seen on imaging scans like X-rays, CT scans, or MRI scans. Solid tumors can occur in different parts of the body, including the breast, lung, colon, prostate, and others.

Liquid tumors, on the other hand, are cancers that affect the blood or lymphatic system. These cancers are also known as leukemias or lymphomas. Leukemias occur when cancer cells affect the bone marrow, where blood cells are produced, while lymphomas affect the lymphatic system, which is part of the immune system.

Tumors can be either benign or malignant. Benign tumors are noncancerous and typically do not pose a significant threat to health. They grow slowly and remain confined to a particular area of the body. In contrast, malignant tumors are cancerous and can grow rapidly, invade nearby tissues, and spread to other parts of the body through the bloodstream or lymphatic system.

The process of cancer spreading from its original site to other parts of the body is known as metastasis. Metastasis occurs when cancer cells break away from the original tumor and travel to other parts of the body through the bloodstream or lymphatic system. Once the cancer cells reach a new site, they can continue to divide and grow, forming new tumors in other parts of the body.

The treatment of tumors in cancer can involve a range of approaches, including surgery, radiation therapy, chemotherapy, targeted therapy, immunotherapy, and hormone therapy. The appropriate treatment for tumors depends on several factors, including the type and stage of cancer, the location of the tumor, and the person's overall health. Early detection and treatment of tumors are critical for improving outcomes and increasing the chances of successful treatment and long-term survival.

In conclusion, tumors are a hallmark of cancer, and understanding the types and characteristics of tumors is critical for the diagnosis and treatment of cancer. While benign tumors are generally noncancerous and do not pose a significant threat to health, malignant tumors can grow rapidly and spread to other parts of the body, making early detection and treatment essential for successful outcomes.

Chapter Two: TYPES OF CANCER

There are many different types of cancer, and they can affect any part of the body. Some of the most common types of cancer include:

Carcinomas:
Carcinomas are the most common type of cancer, accounting for around 80% to 90% of all cancer cases. They start in the epithelial cells, which are the cells that make up the skin or tissues lining internal organs. Carcinomas are further classified into different subtypes based on the type of cell that is affected. For example, squamous cell carcinoma affects the flat cells that make up the skin and the lining of some organs, while adenocarcinoma affects the glandular cells that produce mucus or other fluids.

Sarcomas:
Sarcomas are rare types of cancer that start in the connective tissues of the body, such as bone, cartilage, muscle, or fat. There are two main

types of sarcoma: osteosarcoma, which starts in the bone tissue, and soft tissue sarcoma, which starts in the soft tissues of the body, such as muscle or fat. Sarcomas can be difficult to treat because they often spread quickly to other parts of the body.

Leukemias: Leukemias are cancers that start in the bone marrow, which is the spongy tissue inside bones where blood cells are made. Leukemia cells are abnormal white blood cells that multiply uncontrollably and can crowd out healthy blood cells. There are four main types of leukemia: acute lymphoblastic leukemia (ALL), acute myeloid leukemia (AML), chronic lymphocytic leukemia (CLL), and chronic myeloid leukemia (CML).

Lymphomas:
 Lymphomas are cancers that start in the lymphatic system, which is part of the immune system that helps fight infections. Lymphoma cells are abnormal white blood cells called lymphocytes that multiply uncontrollably and can form tumors in lymph nodes or other parts of the body. There are two main types of

lymphoma: Hodgkin lymphoma and non-Hodgkin lymphoma.

Brain and spinal cord tumors: These are cancers that start in the tissues of the brain or spinal cord. There are many different types of brain and spinal cord tumors, and they are named based on the type of cell they start in, as well as other characteristics such as their location and how quickly they grow. Some common types of brain and spinal cord tumors include gliomas, meningiomas, and astrocytomas.

Germ cell tumors:
Germ cell tumors are cancers that start in the cells that produce sperm or eggs. These tumors can occur in the testicles or ovaries, as well as other parts of the body such as the chest or abdomen. There are two main types of germ cell tumors: seminomas and non-seminomas.

Neuroendocrine tumors:
Neuroendocrine tumors are cancers that start in cells that produce hormones. These tumors can occur in various parts of the body, such as

the pancreas, intestines, or lungs. They can be benign or malignant, and treatment depends on several factors such as the size and location of the tumor.

Mesothelioma:
 Mesothelioma is a rare type of cancer that starts in the lining of the lungs, abdomen, or heart. It is often caused by exposure to asbestos, which is a mineral that was commonly used in construction and other industries before its health hazards were recognized. Mesothelioma is often difficult to diagnose and treat, and the prognosis is generally poor.

It's important to note that there are many other types of cancer as well, and each type can have different subtypes and variations. The appropriate treatment for each type of cancer depends on several factors, including the stage of the cancer, the location

Symptoms and possible treatment

Carcinomas:

Symptoms: Symptoms of carcinomas can vary
depending on the type and location of the
cancer. Common symptoms may include a
lump or thickening in the skin or tissue,
changes in skin color or texture, persistent
cough or hoarseness, difficulty swallowing,
changes in bowel or bladder habits, and
unexplained weight loss.
Treatments: Treatment options for carcinomas
may include surgery, radiation therapy,
chemotherapy, targeted therapy, and
immunotherapy. The appropriate treatment
will depend on the type and stage of the cancer.

Sarcomas:
Symptoms: Symptoms of sarcomas may include
a lump or swelling in the affected area, pain or
discomfort, limited range of motion, and
weakness or numbness in the affected limb.
Treatments: Treatment options for sarcomas
may include surgery, radiation therapy,
chemotherapy, and targeted therapy. The
appropriate treatment will depend on the type,
location, and stage of the cancer.

Leukemias:

Symptoms: Symptoms of leukemias may include fatigue, weakness, pale skin, frequent infections, fever, easy bleeding or bruising, swollen lymph nodes, and bone pain.
Treatments: Treatment options for leukemias may include chemotherapy, targeted therapy, radiation therapy, stem cell transplant, and immunotherapy. The appropriate treatment will depend on the type and stage of the leukemia.

Lymphomas:
Symptoms: Symptoms of lymphomas may include swollen lymph nodes, fever, night sweats, unexplained weight loss, fatigue, and itching.
Treatments: Treatment options for lymphomas may include chemotherapy, radiation therapy, targeted therapy, stem cell transplant, and immunotherapy. The appropriate treatment will depend on the type, stage, and location of the cancer.

Brain and spinal cord tumors:
Symptoms: Symptoms of brain and spinal cord tumors may include headaches, seizures,

difficulty thinking or speaking, changes in vision, weakness or numbness in the limbs, and balance problems.
Treatments: Treatment options for brain and spinal cord tumors may include surgery, radiation therapy, chemotherapy, and targeted therapy. The appropriate treatment will depend on the type, location, and stage of the tumor.

Germ cell tumors:
Symptoms: Symptoms of germ cell tumors may include a lump or swelling in the testicles or ovaries, abdominal pain or swelling, and unexplained weight loss.
Treatments: Treatment options for germ cell tumors may include surgery, chemotherapy, radiation therapy, and targeted therapy. The appropriate treatment will depend on the type, location, and stage of the tumor.

Neuroendocrine tumors:
Symptoms: Symptoms of neuroendocrine tumors may vary depending on the location and type of the tumor. Common symptoms may include abdominal pain, diarrhea, flushing, wheezing, and weight loss.

Treatments: Treatment options for neuroendocrine tumors may include surgery, chemotherapy, radiation therapy, and targeted therapy. The appropriate treatment will depend on the type, location, and stage of the tumor.

Mesothelioma:
Symptoms: Symptoms of mesothelioma may include shortness of breath, chest pain, cough, fatigue, and weight loss.
Treatments: Treatment options for mesothelioma may include surgery, chemotherapy, radiation therapy, and targeted therapy. The appropriate treatment will depend on the stage, location, and extent of the cancer.

It's important to note that the symptoms and treatments for each type of cancer can vary widely, and each case should be evaluated and treated on an individual basis by a qualified healthcare professional. So if you notice anything out of the ordinary rush to do a check up at a certified Hospital with qualified doctors

Some of the most dangerous types of cancer

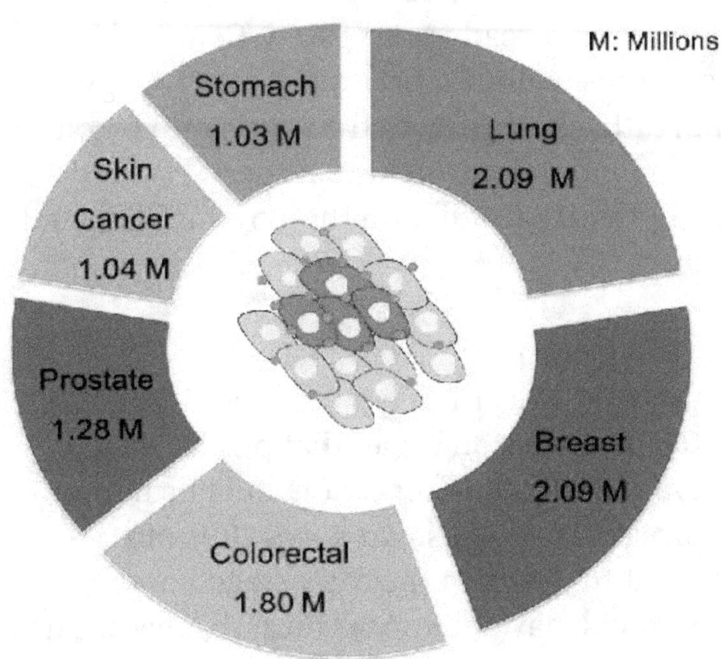

The most dangerous types of cancer are those that are associated with a high mortality rate and can be difficult to treat. Some of the most dangerous types of cancer include:

Lung cancer:
 Lung cancer is a malignant tumor that starts in the lungs. The majority of lung cancers are caused by smoking or exposure to secondhand smoke, and symptoms may not appear until the disease has already progressed. Common symptoms include a persistent cough, shortness of breath, chest pain, and coughing up blood. Treatment options include surgery, chemotherapy, radiation therapy, and targeted therapy.

Pancreatic cancer:
Pancreatic cancer is a type of cancer that starts in the pancreas, an organ that produces enzymes that aid in digestion and hormones that regulate blood sugar levels. It is often difficult to detect in the early stages, and symptoms may not appear until the disease has already spread to other organs. Common symptoms include abdominal pain, weight loss, jaundice, and nausea. Treatment options include surgery, chemotherapy, radiation therapy, and targeted therapy.

Liver cancer:

Liver cancer is a type of cancer that starts in the liver, an organ that plays a vital role in the digestive system and other bodily functions. It is often associated with chronic liver disease or heavy alcohol use, and symptoms may not appear until the disease has progressed to a more advanced stage. Common symptoms include abdominal pain, weight loss, fatigue, and yellowing of the skin and eyes. Treatment options include surgery, chemotherapy, radiation therapy, and targeted therapy.

Colorectal cancer:
 Colorectal cancer is a type of cancer that starts in the colon or rectum, and is often diagnosed in older adults. It can develop from polyps, which are growths in the colon or rectum. Common symptoms include changes in bowel habits, blood in the stool, abdominal pain, and weight loss. Treatment options include surgery, chemotherapy, radiation therapy, and targeted therapy.

Breast cancer:
Breast cancer is a type of cancer that starts in the breast tissue, and is the most common

cancer among women worldwide. It can develop in both men and women, but is more common in women. Common symptoms include a lump or thickening in the breast tissue, changes in the size or shape of the breast, nipple discharge, and skin changes. Treatment options include surgery, chemotherapy, radiation therapy, and targeted therapy.

Prostate cancer:
Prostate cancer is a type of cancer that starts in the prostate gland, which is located in the male reproductive system. It is often diagnosed in older men, and can develop slowly over many years. Common symptoms include difficulty urinating, frequent urination, blood in the urine, and pain in the lower back, hips, or thighs. Treatment options include surgery, radiation therapy, hormone therapy, and chemotherapy.

Ovarian cancer:
Ovarian cancer is a type of cancer that starts in the ovaries, which are part of the female reproductive system. It is often diagnosed in

later stages, when it has already spread to other parts of the body. Common symptoms include abdominal pain, bloating, changes in bowel habits, and urinary urgency. Treatment options include surgery, chemotherapy, radiation therapy, and targeted therapy.

It's important to remember that every individual's cancer diagnosis and treatment plan is unique, and should be discussed with a medical professional. Early detection and prompt treatment can greatly improve the chances of successful recovery.

CAUSES OF CANCER

Cancer is a complex disease that can be caused by a variety of factors. Here are some known causes of cancer:

Genetic mutations: Cancer can be caused by changes or mutations in the DNA of cells. These mutations can be inherited or acquired, and they can occur due to various factors, such as exposure to environmental toxins, radiation, and viral infections. Inherited mutations account for a small percentage of all cancers, while acquired mutations are more common and are often related to lifestyle factors.

Environmental factors: Exposure to certain chemicals, toxins, radiation, and pollutants can increase the risk of cancer. For example, prolonged exposure to asbestos fibers can increase the risk of developing lung cancer, mesothelioma, and other types of cancer. Exposure to ultraviolet (UV) radiation from the sun or tanning beds can increase the risk of skin cancer. Air pollution, including particulate matter and diesel exhaust, has been linked to lung cancer, as well as other types of cancer.

Lifestyle factors: Certain habits and behaviors can contribute to the development of cancer. Smoking tobacco is the leading cause of lung cancer, but it is also a risk factor for many other types of cancer, including bladder, kidney, and pancreatic cancer. Excessive alcohol consumption has been linked to an increased risk of liver, colorectal, and breast cancer. A poor diet, which is high in processed and red meat, unhealthy fats, and low in fruits and vegetables, can also increase the risk of cancer. Lack of physical activity and obesity are also risk factors for several types of cancer.

Viral infections: Some viruses can increase the risk of developing cancer. For example, human papillomavirus (HPV) is a sexually transmitted virus that can cause cervical, anal, and other types of cancer. Hepatitis B and C viruses can cause liver cancer. Human immunodeficiency virus (HIV) weakens the immune system, increasing the risk of developing several types of cancer.

Age: Cancer can occur at any age, but the risk of developing cancer increases as people get older. This is because DNA damage accumulates over time, and the immune system becomes less effective at detecting and eliminating cancer cells.

Family history: Certain types of cancer can be caused by inherited genetic mutations. For example, mutations in the BRCA1 and BRCA2 genes can increase the risk of developing breast and ovarian cancer. Other types of cancer, such as colon cancer, can also have a genetic component, and people with a family history of these cancers may be at a higher risk of developing the disease.

In summary, cancer is a complex disease that can be caused by a combination of genetic, environmental, lifestyle, and other factors. While not all cancers can be prevented, reducing exposure to known risk factors and maintaining a healthy lifestyle can help reduce the risk of developing cancer.

Chapter Three: STAGES OF CANCER

Cancer is often described in stages that reflect how far the disease has progressed. The stages of cancer are based on the size and location of the tumor, whether it has spread to nearby lymph nodes or other parts of the body, and other factors specific to the type of cancer. The following is a general overview of the different stages of cancer:

Stage 0:
This stage is also known as carcinoma in situ. The cancerous cells are confined to the layer of cells where they first developed and have not spread to nearby tissue. At this stage, the cancer is highly treatable, and most people are cured with surgery or other local treatments.

Stage I:
At this stage, the cancer is small and has not spread to nearby lymph nodes or other parts of the body. The tumor is typically less than 2 cm in size, and there is no evidence of cancer in nearby lymph nodes or organs. Depending on the type of cancer, treatment may involve surgery, radiation therapy, or a combination of both.

Stage II:

At this stage, the cancer has grown larger and may have spread to nearby lymph nodes, but it has not yet spread to distant parts of the body. The tumor may be larger than 2 cm, or it may have grown into nearby tissues or organs. Treatment typically involves a combination of surgery, radiation therapy, and chemotherapy.

Stage III:
At this stage, the cancer has grown larger and has spread to nearby lymph nodes and possibly other nearby tissues or organs. The tumor may have invaded nearby blood vessels or organs. Treatment may involve surgery, radiation therapy, chemotherapy, or a combination of these treatments.

Stage IV:
At this stage, the cancer has spread to distant parts of the body, such as the lungs, liver, or bones. This is also called metastatic cancer. Treatment may involve surgery, radiation therapy, chemotherapy, targeted therapy, immunotherapy, or a combination of these treatments. The goal of treatment at this stage is usually to manage symptoms, improve

quality of life, and slow the progression of the disease.

In addition to these general stages, some cancers have specific sub-stages that provide more detail about the extent of the disease. For example, breast cancer is often described using the TNM system, which takes into account the size of the tumor (T), whether it has spread to nearby lymph nodes (N), and whether it has metastasized (M) to other parts of the body. The TNM system also includes sub-stages based on the number and location of affected lymph nodes.

It's important to note that cancer staging is specific to each type of cancer and can be quite complex. The stage of cancer is important in determining the appropriate treatment options and prognosis. Your doctor can provide more information about the stage of your cancer and what it means for your treatment options and outlook.

TREATMENTS FOR CANCER

These are some of the options available for treating cancer

Surgery:
 Surgery is often the first treatment option for cancer. It involves removing the tumor and surrounding tissue, with the goal of removing all the cancerous cells. Surgery can be curative in some cases, particularly when the cancer is caught early and has not spread to other parts of the body. Surgery may be followed by other treatments, such as chemotherapy or radiation therapy, to help prevent the cancer from returning.

Radiation therapy:
Radiation therapy uses high-energy radiation, such as X-rays or protons, to kill cancer cells. The radiation is targeted at the tumor, with the goal of destroying as many cancer cells as possible while minimizing damage to healthy tissue. Radiation therapy can be used as the primary treatment for some cancers, or it can be used in combination with other treatments, such as surgery or chemotherapy.

Chemotherapy:
Chemotherapy uses drugs to kill cancer cells throughout the body. The drugs are typically given by injection or taken orally, and they circulate throughout the bloodstream, targeting cancer cells wherever they may be. Chemotherapy can be used as the primary treatment for some cancers, or it can be used in combination with other treatments, such as surgery or radiation therapy. Chemotherapy is often associated with side effects, such as nausea, hair loss, and fatigue, but newer treatments have helped to reduce these side effects.

Immunotherapy:
A Immunotherapy is a type of cancer treatment that harnesses the power of the immune system to fight cancer. It involves stimulating the immune system to recognize and attack cancer cells, either by boosting the body's natural immune response or by using synthetic antibodies or other immune system components. Immunotherapy can be used as the primary treatment for some cancers, or it can be used in combination with other

treatments, such as chemotherapy or radiation therapy. Immunotherapy is often associated with fewer side effects than other cancer treatments.

Other types of cancer treatments include targeted therapy, hormone therapy, and stem cell transplant. Targeted therapy uses drugs to target specific molecules or proteins that are involved in cancer growth, while hormone therapy is used to treat cancers that are sensitive to hormones, such as breast cancer or prostate cancer. Stem cell transplant involves replacing the patient's diseased bone marrow with healthy stem cells, which can help to rebuild the immune system and fight cancer.

The choice of treatment depends on several factors, such as the type and stage of cancer, the patient's overall health, and their personal preferences. Your doctor can provide more information about the available treatment options and which ones may be most appropriate for you.

Part two

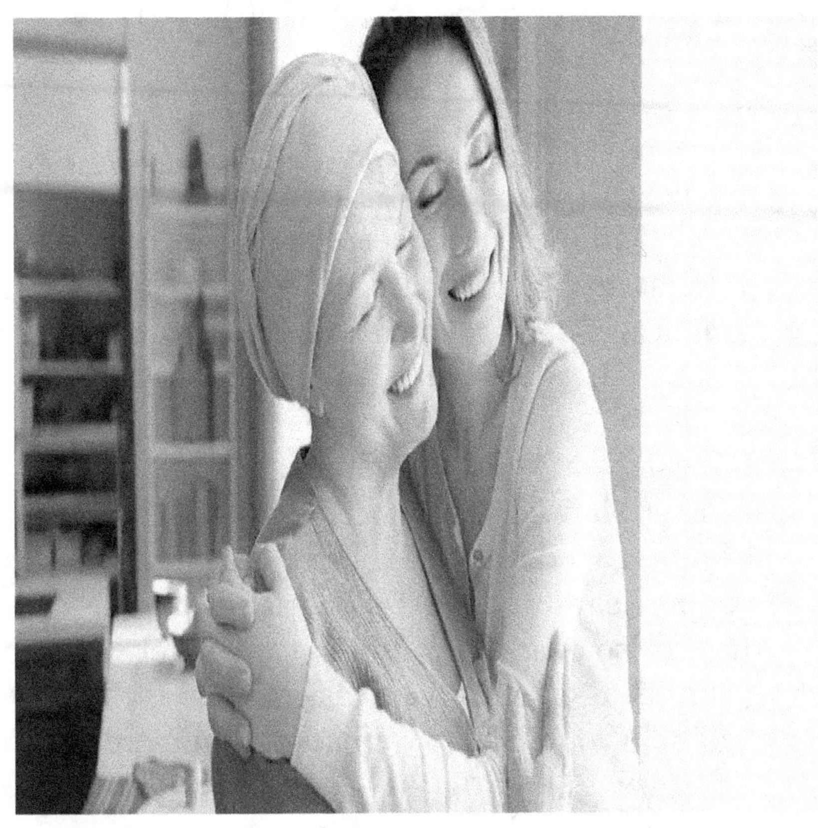

Chapter four: LIVING WITH CANCER

Living with cancer can be a challenging and overwhelming experience, but there are many ways to manage the physical, emotional, and practical aspects of the disease. Here are some tips to help you cope:

Educate yourself about cancer:
 Understanding your cancer diagnosis, the stage of cancer, and the available treatments can help you make informed decisions about your care. It can also help you communicate better with your healthcare team and ask questions that will help you manage your condition more effectively.

Build a support system:
Coping with cancer can be emotionally and physically challenging. Reach out to family, friends, or support groups for emotional

support, practical help with daily activities, or even just someone to talk to. Support groups can also connect you with others who understand what you're going through and offer helpful tips and advice.

Take care of your body:
 Eating a healthy diet, staying physically active, and getting enough sleep can help your body cope with cancer treatment and reduce side effects. Exercise can also boost your mood and help you feel more energized.

Manage your stress:
Cancer can cause significant stress and anxiety. Finding ways to manage stress, such as meditation, mindfulness, or yoga, can help you cope better with the emotional and physical challenges of cancer. Consider talking to a therapist or counselor who specializes in working with people with cancer.

Stay organized:
Keep track of your appointments, medications, and side effects. This can help you stay on top of your treatment plan and feel more in control

of your care. Consider using a planner or app to help you stay organized.

Be kind to yourself:
Cancer can take a toll on your emotional and physical well-being. Give yourself permission to rest when you need it, and take time for activities that you enjoy. This can help you feel more refreshed and better able to cope with the challenges of cancer.

Stay positive:
Maintaining a positive outlook can help you feel more hopeful and resilient. Focus on the things that bring you joy and gratitude, and try to find ways to stay engaged with activities and people you love. Remember that it's okay to feel sad, angry, or frustrated at times, but staying positive can help you cope better with the challenges of cancer.

These are just a few suggestions to help you cope with cancer. Remember that everyone's experience is different, and it's important to find what works best for you. Don't hesitate to

reach out to your healthcare team or a
counselor if you need additional support.

Chapter Five: DEALING WITH EMOTIONAL AND PHYSICAL IMPACTS OF CANCER

Managing the emotional and physical impact of cancer can be challenging, but there are several strategies that can help:

Seek support:
Having a strong support network can help you manage the emotional and physical impact of cancer. Your support network may include family and friends who can provide emotional support, help you with practical tasks, and accompany you to appointments. You may also find it helpful to connect with others who are going through a similar experience, such as joining a support group or online community. Additionally, a therapist or counselor who specializes in cancer-related issues can provide you with tools to manage stress, anxiety, and other emotional issues.

Take care of your physical health:
Taking care of your physical health can help you
manage the physical impact of cancer. Eating a
healthy diet that includes a variety of fruits,
vegetables, whole grains, and lean proteins can
help you maintain your strength and energy.
Exercise can also help improve your physical
well-being and can be tailored to your
individual needs and abilities. Additionally, it's
important to take medication as prescribed by
your healthcare provider, and to manage any
side effects you may experience.

Practice self-care:
 Self-care practices can help you manage both
the emotional and physical impact of cancer.
Engaging in activities that you enjoy can help
you maintain a sense of normalcy and can
improve your mood. Taking time to relax can
help reduce stress and anxiety, and
participating in complementary therapies such
as massage or acupuncture can help manage
physical symptoms. Engaging in creative
activities such as art or music can also be a
helpful way to manage your emotions and
express yourself.

Communicate with your healthcare team:
 Your healthcare team can provide you with
information about treatment options, support
services, and symptom management strategies.
It's important to communicate with them about
any physical symptoms or emotional issues you
may be experiencing so that they can provide
you with the best possible care.

Manage your stress:
Stress can have a significant impact on your
emotional and physical well-being. Engaging in
relaxation techniques such as deep breathing
exercises, meditation, or yoga can help you
manage your stress levels. Participating in
physical activities such as walking, swimming,
or dancing can also be an effective way to
manage stress.

Educate yourself:
Learning as much as you can about your
diagnosis, treatment options, and prognosis can
help you feel more in control and less anxious.
Your healthcare team can provide you with
resources, and there are also organizations that

provide information and support to people living with cancer.

Remember, coping with the emotional and physical impact of cancer is a journey. It's important to be patient with yourself and to seek support when you need it. With the right strategies and support, you can manage your symptoms and improve your overall well-being.

Chapter Six: HOW TO DEAL WITH CHANGES FROM TAKING TREATMENTS

Dealing with the effects of cancer treatment can be a challenging and emotional experience. Depending on the type of cancer and the treatment plan, you may experience a variety of physical and emotional changes. Here are some additional strategies that may help:

Talk to your healthcare team:
Your healthcare team is a valuable resource for information and support. They can help you understand the side effects of your treatment and suggest strategies to manage them. Your healthcare team may also be able to adjust your treatment plan to minimize side effects or recommend other therapies to alleviate symptoms.

Practice self-care:
Taking care of yourself during cancer treatment is important for your overall well-being. Eat a healthy diet with plenty of fruits and vegetables,

whole grains, and lean proteins. Get enough sleep each night and aim to exercise regularly, as advised by your healthcare team. Exercise can help reduce fatigue, improve mood, and increase overall well-being. Additionally, take time to engage in activities you enjoy and find relaxing, such as reading, spending time with loved ones, or practicing meditation.

Manage side effects:
 There are many strategies to manage specific side effects of cancer treatment, such as nausea, pain, and neuropathy. Your healthcare team may recommend medications or complementary therapies, such as acupuncture or massage, to help manage these symptoms. Additionally, lifestyle changes such as eating small, frequent meals or using heat or cold therapy may also be helpful.

Seek support:
Cancer treatment can be emotionally taxing, and it's important to seek support from family, friends, or a counselor. Joining a support group or speaking with a counselor can help you cope with the emotional impact of cancer treatment.

Additionally, your healthcare team may be able to recommend resources in your community.

Stay informed:
Learning as much as you can about your treatment and its potential side effects can help you feel more in control and better prepared to manage any changes that occur. Ask your healthcare team questions and keep a record of any side effects you experience. This can help you track your symptoms and communicate more effectively with your healthcare team.

Remember that everyone's experience with cancer treatment is unique, and what works for one person may not work for another. Be patient with yourself and don't hesitate to reach out to your healthcare team for guidance and support. With time and care, many people are able to manage the effects of cancer treatment and continue to live full and meaningful lives.

EATING HEALTHY FOODS

When it comes to a healthy diet for a cancer patient, it's important to focus on nutrient-dense foods that can help support the immune system and promote overall health. Here are some examples of healthy foods and dietary patterns for cancer patients:

Fruits and vegetables:
 Fruits and vegetables are rich in antioxidants, vitamins, and minerals that can help protect the body against cancer and promote healing. Aim for a variety of colorful produce, such as leafy greens, berries, citrus fruits, tomatoes, carrots, and sweet potatoes.

Whole grains:
Whole grains are a good source of fiber and other important nutrients that can help regulate digestion and blood sugar levels. Examples of whole grains include brown rice, quinoa, whole wheat bread, and oatmeal.

Lean protein:
Protein is important for maintaining muscle mass and promoting healing, but it's important to choose lean sources to avoid excess saturated fat. Good options include skinless chicken or turkey, fish, beans, lentils, and tofu.

Healthy fats:
Healthy fats, such as those found in nuts, seeds, avocados, and olive oil, can help reduce inflammation and support overall health.

In addition to these healthy foods, there are also some dietary patterns that may be particularly beneficial for cancer patients. For example, the Mediterranean diet, which emphasizes whole grains, fruits and vegetables, lean protein, and healthy fats, has been linked to a lower risk of cancer and improved outcomes in cancer patients. The DASH (Dietary Approaches to Stop Hypertension) diet, which focuses on fruits and vegetables, whole grains, and low-fat dairy products, may also be beneficial for cancer patients, particularly those who have hypertension.

It's important to work with a registered dietitian or healthcare provider to develop an individualized nutrition plan that takes into account your specific needs and treatment plan.

Eating a healthy diet, exercising regularly, getting enough sleep, and incorporating complementary therapies like meditation and acupuncture can be incredibly beneficial for cancer patients. Here's why:

Healthy Diet:
A healthy diet can help cancer patients maintain a healthy weight, boost their immune system, and reduce inflammation in the body. Eating a diet rich in fruits, vegetables, whole grains, lean protein, and healthy fats can provide the necessary nutrients that the body needs to function at its best. Additionally, some foods have been shown to have anti-cancer properties, such as cruciferous vegetables like

broccoli and cauliflower, which contain compounds that may help prevent cancer.

Exercise:
Regular exercise can help cancer patients manage their symptoms and improve their overall quality of life. Exercise can reduce fatigue, improve mood, and boost energy levels. It can also help patients maintain their muscle mass and bone density, which is especially important for those undergoing chemotherapy, which can cause muscle weakness and bone loss.

Sleep:
Getting enough restful sleep is crucial for cancer patients. During sleep, the body repairs and regenerates damaged tissues, and the immune system is strengthened. Lack of sleep can weaken the immune system and increase inflammation in the body, which can make it harder for cancer patients to fight off infections and recover from treatments.

Complementary Therapies:
Complementary therapies like meditation and acupuncture can help cancer patients manage their symptoms and improve their quality of life. Meditation can reduce anxiety and stress, improve sleep quality, and boost the immune system. Acupuncture can help relieve pain, reduce nausea and vomiting, and improve overall well-being.

In summary, eating a healthy diet, exercising regularly, getting enough sleep, and incorporating complementary therapies like meditation and acupuncture can be incredibly beneficial for cancer patients. They can help manage symptoms, boost the immune system, improve quality of life, and potentially even improve outcomes. It's important to talk to a healthcare provider before starting any new exercise or complementary therapy regimen to ensure safety and efficacy.

Part Three

Chapter Seven: Building support network

A support network can be incredibly beneficial for people who are dealing with cancer. A cancer diagnosis can be a very difficult and emotional experience, and having a support network can help patients cope with the physical, emotional, and psychological challenges of the disease.

A support network can include family members, friends, healthcare professionals, and support groups. Family members and friends can provide emotional support, help with daily tasks, and offer encouragement and motivation. Healthcare professionals, such as doctors, nurses, and counselors, can provide medical support, information about treatment options, and emotional support. Support groups can provide patients with the opportunity to connect with others who are going through similar experiences, share information and advice, and provide emotional support.

Studies have shown that having a strong support network can improve the quality of life for cancer patients, increase their ability to cope with the disease, and improve their overall health outcomes. For example, research has shown that cancer patients with social support are less likely to experience depression and anxiety, and have a better overall quality of life.

In addition, a support network can also provide practical help and assistance to cancer patients, such as helping with transportation to medical appointments, preparing meals, and taking care of children or pets.

Overall, a strong support network can be an important factor in helping cancer patients cope with the physical, emotional, and psychological challenges of the disease, and can ultimately lead to better health outcomes.

SUPPORT NETWORK OF FRIENDS

Having a support network of friends can be especially important for cancer patients. Friends can provide emotional support, practical help, and a sense of normalcy during a difficult time.

Emotional support from friends can include offering a listening ear, providing words of encouragement and motivation, and simply being there to offer comfort and companionship. Studies have shown that cancer patients who have social support from friends have better mental health outcomes and experience less distress and anxiety.

Friends can also offer practical help to cancer patients, such as providing transportation to medical appointments, preparing meals, running errands, and taking care of household tasks. This kind of practical support can be especially important for patients who are undergoing treatment and may have limited energy and mobility.

In addition, friends can provide a sense of normalcy and help patients maintain a social life and stay connected to their communities. Cancer treatment can be isolating, and having a support network of friends can help patients maintain a sense of identity and purpose outside of their illness.

It's important for cancer patients to communicate their needs and preferences to their friends, and for friends to be responsive and willing to help. Friends can also be encouraged to educate themselves about the patient's diagnosis and treatment options, so they can better understand what the patient is going through and provide appropriate support.

Overall, a support network of friends can be an invaluable resource for cancer patients, providing emotional support, practical help, and a sense of normalcy during a challenging time.

SUPPORT NETWORK OF HEALTHCARE PROFESSIONALS

A support network of healthcare professionals refers to a group of individuals within the healthcare industry who provide support to one another. This can be in the form of emotional support, professional development, or sharing of knowledge and expertise.

In the healthcare industry, healthcare professionals work in demanding and often stressful environments. Having a support network of colleagues who understand the challenges of the job and can provide support can be crucial for maintaining good mental health and avoiding burnout.

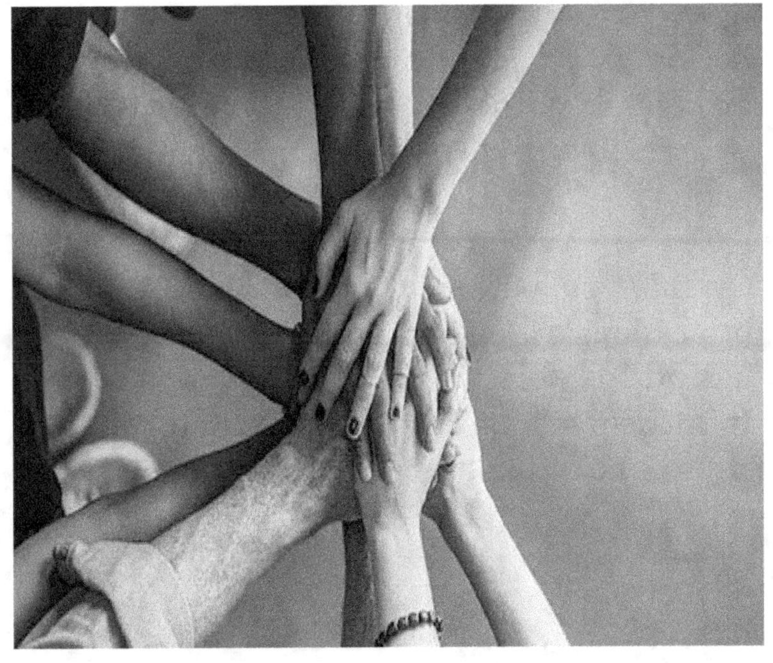

Some examples of healthcare professionals who may form a support network include nurses, doctors, therapists, social workers, and other allied health professionals. These individuals may connect through professional organizations, online forums, or in-person support groups.

In addition to providing emotional support, a support network of healthcare professionals can also offer opportunities for professional development and collaboration. For example, doctors may share their expertise with nurses, and therapists may collaborate with social workers to provide comprehensive care for patients.

Overall, a support network of healthcare professionals is an important resource for individuals working in the healthcare industry. It can help to improve job satisfaction, reduce stress, and ultimately lead to better patient care.

Chapter Eight: FINDING YOUR SUPPORT GROUP

Finding a support group during your cancer journey can be a valuable source of emotional support and a safe space to share your experiences with others who are going through similar challenges. Here are some steps you can take to find a support group:

Talk to your healthcare team:
Your healthcare team may have information on support groups in your area, or they may be able to refer you to a social worker who can provide additional resources.

Use online resources:
There are several websites and forums dedicated to connecting people with cancer support groups. Some examples include the American Cancer Society's Cancer Survivors Network, CancerCare, and the Cancer Support Community.

Reach out to local organizations:

Check with local hospitals, community centers, or cancer advocacy organizations to see if they offer support groups.

Ask other cancer survivors:
If you know someone who has gone through cancer treatment, ask them if they know of any support groups that may be helpful for you.

Once you have found a support group, it is important to advocate for yourself throughout your cancer journey. Here are some tips:

Educate yourself:
Learn as much as you can about your cancer diagnosis, treatment options, and any side effects or complications that may arise. This knowledge will help you make informed decisions about your care.

Speak up:
If you have questions or concerns about your treatment plan, don't be afraid to speak up and ask your healthcare team for clarification or more information.

Keep track of your symptoms:
 Keep a record of any symptoms or side effects
you experience during your treatment, and
bring them to your healthcare team's attention.
This can help them adjust your treatment plan
as needed.

Seek a second opinion:
If you are unsure about your treatment plan or
diagnosis, don't hesitate to seek a second
opinion from another healthcare provider.

Connect with advocacy organizations:
There are several cancer advocacy organizations
that can provide resources and support to help
you advocate for yourself throughout your
cancer journey. Some examples include the
American Cancer Society, CancerCare, and the
National Cancer Institute.

BENEFITS OF SUPPORT GROUPS

Having a support group during your cancer
journey can offer a wide range of benefits,
including:

Emotional support:
A support group can provide a safe and supportive space where you can share your feelings, fears, and concerns with others who are going through similar experiences. This can help alleviate feelings of isolation and loneliness and promote a sense of community.

Information and resources:
Support groups can provide valuable information and resources about cancer treatments, side effects, and coping strategies. This can help you make informed decisions about your care and improve your overall quality of life.

Peer validation:
 Hearing from others who are going through similar experiences can help validate your feelings and experiences, which can be especially important when dealing with the emotional toll of a cancer diagnosis.

Improved coping skills:
Support groups can help you learn effective coping strategies for managing stress, anxiety,

and other emotional challenges associated with cancer.

Sense of empowerment:
Connecting with others who have experienced cancer can help you feel more empowered and in control of your cancer journey.

Sense of hope:
Being part of a support group can help instill a sense of hope and optimism, as you see others who have successfully navigated their cancer journey and are living fulfilling lives.

Overall, a support group can provide a valuable source of emotional support and practical information, helping you navigate the challenges of cancer treatment and recovery.

Part Four

Chapter Nine: LIVING WITH UNCERTAINTY

Cancer is a disease that can bring a lot of uncertainty and anxiety for both the patient and their loved ones. There are many unknown factors when it comes to cancer, including the cause of the disease, how it will progress, and how it will respond to treatment. This uncertainty can be particularly challenging, as it can be difficult to plan for the future and make important decisions.

One of the best ways to deal with uncertainty in the face of cancer is to stay informed. This means working closely with healthcare professionals to understand the disease, the available treatments, and the potential outcomes. It's also important to stay connected with loved ones, who can offer emotional support and help with practical matters.

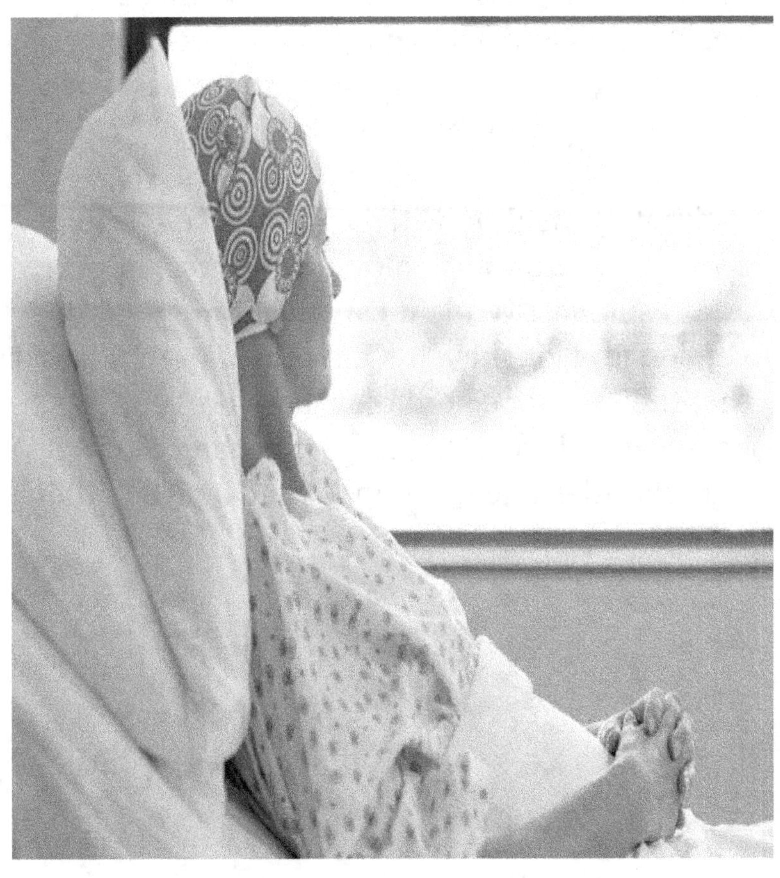

Another important strategy is to focus on what can be controlled. While it's true that there are many unknowns when it comes to cancer, there are also many things that can be done to manage the disease and its symptoms. This may include lifestyle changes, such as eating a healthy diet and getting regular exercise, as well as seeking out complementary therapies, such as acupuncture or meditation.

Ultimately, dealing with cancer and uncertainty requires a combination of knowledge, support, and resilience. While it can be a difficult and challenging journey, it's important to remember that there is hope, and that there are many people who have successfully navigated the uncertainties of cancer and come out the other side.

Chapter Ten: HELPFUL TIPS AFTER RECEIVING NEWS OF CANCER

Receiving a cancer diagnosis can be a challenging and overwhelming experience, and it is natural to feel anxious, fearful, or uncertain about the future. However, it is possible to stay present in the moment, find joy and meaning in life, and cope with the challenges of cancer by following these tips:

Practice mindfulness:
 Mindfulness involves being present in the moment, without judgment or distraction. Mindfulness practices such as meditation, deep breathing exercises, and yoga can help to reduce stress, improve mental clarity, and increase overall well-being.

Connect with others:
Building and maintaining social connections with friends, family, and support groups can help to reduce feelings of isolation and

loneliness, and provide a sense of belonging and purpose.

Engage in meaningful activities:
 Finding activities that bring joy and purpose, such as hobbies, volunteering, or spending time in nature, can help to improve mood and provide a sense of fulfillment and meaning.

Take care of your physical health:
Maintaining a healthy diet, getting regular exercise, and following medical treatment plans can help to improve physical health, reduce symptoms, and increase energy levels.

Seek professional support:
Working with a therapist, counselor, or other mental health professional can provide additional support and guidance for coping with the emotional and psychological challenges of cancer.

Focus on gratitude:
Practicing gratitude, such as keeping a gratitude journal or reflecting on the positive aspects of life, can help to cultivate a sense of

appreciation and resilience, even during
difficult times.

Practice self-compassion:
 Cancer can be a difficult and emotional
journey, and it is important to practice
self-compassion and kindness towards yourself.
This involves treating yourself with the same
care and understanding that you would offer to
a good friend or loved one.

Engage in creative expression:
Engaging in creative activities such as painting,
writing, or music can be a powerful way to
express emotions, find joy, and explore new
ways of thinking.

Connect with nature:
Spending time in nature, whether it is a walk in
the park or a hike in the mountains, can help to
reduce stress and increase feelings of calmness
and relaxation.

Set small goals:
Setting achievable goals, such as completing a puzzle or reading a book, can provide a sense of accomplishment and boost self-esteem.

Practice relaxation techniques:
Relaxation techniques such as progressive muscle relaxation, visualization, or guided imagery can help to reduce stress and promote feelings of relaxation and calmness.

Find meaning in your experiences:
Reflecting on the meaning and purpose of your experiences, and finding ways to incorporate these experiences into a larger narrative of your life, can help to create a sense of coherence and meaning.

Remember, coping with cancer is a personal journey, and what works for one person may not work for another. It is important to explore different options and find the strategies that work best for you. Additionally, working with your healthcare team to manage symptoms and side effects, and following recommended treatment plans, can help to improve physical health and increase feelings of well-being. Receiving a cancer diagnosis can be a challenging and overwhelming experience, and it is natural to feel anxious, fearful, or uncertain about the future. However, it is possible to stay present in the moment, find joy and meaning in life, and cope with the challenges of cancer

Chapter Eleven: MAINTAINING HOPE AND RESILIENCE

Maintaining hope and resilience in the face of uncertainty is an important part of coping with cancer. Here are some tips for cultivating hope and resilience:

Stay informed:
 Learn as much as you can about your diagnosis and treatment options. Staying informed can help to reduce anxiety and provide a sense of control.

Practice self-care:
 Take care of your physical, emotional, and spiritual needs. This can include exercise, healthy eating, stress management, and relaxation techniques.

Build a support network:
Seek out support from friends, family, and healthcare professionals. Joining a support group or speaking with a therapist can also be helpful.

Cultivate a positive mindset:
Try to focus on the positive aspects of your life, such as relationships, hobbies, and accomplishments. This can help to reduce negative thinking and promote a sense of optimism.

Set goals and celebrate accomplishments:
Setting achievable goals and celebrating even small accomplishments can provide a sense of purpose and boost self-esteem.

Practice gratitude:
Focus on the things in your life that you are grateful for, such as relationships, experiences, and personal strengths. This can help to cultivate a sense of appreciation and resilience.

Take one day at a time:
Coping with cancer can be overwhelming, and it is important to take things one day at a time. Try to focus on the present moment and what you can do to take care of yourself today.

Engage in activities that bring you joy:
Engaging in activities that bring you pleasure, such as spending time with loved ones, listening to music, or reading, can help to boost your mood and increase feelings of well-being.

Practice mindfulness:
Mindfulness practices such as meditation, deep breathing exercises, and yoga can help to reduce stress, improve mental clarity, and increase overall well-being.

Seek out role models:
Connecting with others who have coped with cancer and emerged stronger can provide inspiration and a sense of hope. Look for support groups or online communities where you can connect with others who have similar experiences.

Stay connected with your healthcare team:
Regular check-ins with your healthcare team can help you stay informed about your treatment progress and any changes in your condition. It can also provide a sense of support and guidance.

Find meaning in your experience:
Reflecting on the meaning and purpose of your experiences, and finding ways to incorporate these experiences into a larger narrative of your life, can help to create a sense of coherence and meaning.

Maintain a sense of humor:
 Humor can be a powerful coping mechanism, and finding ways to laugh and see the lighter side of things can help to reduce stress and promote a sense of positivity

Remember, maintaining hope and resilience is a process, and it is normal to experience ups and downs along the way.

Part Five

Chapter Twelve: PLANNING THE FUTURE

Planning for the future when facing a cancer diagnosis can be challenging, but it is important to consider your options and make decisions that feel right for you. Here are some things to consider when planning for the future with cancer:

Talk to your healthcare team:
 Your healthcare team can provide information about your treatment options and how they may impact your future. This can help you make informed decisions about your care.

Consider your priorities:
 Think about what is most important to you, such as spending time with loved ones, pursuing a particular goal, or maintaining a certain quality of life. This can help you make

decisions about your treatment and other aspects of your life.

Make legal and financial arrangements: Consider creating a will or advance directive, and make sure that your financial affairs are in order. You may also want to consider long-term care options or disability insurance.

Seek out support: Consider joining a support group or speaking with a counselor or therapist. These resources can provide emotional support and help you navigate the challenges of planning for the future.

Focus on the present: While it is important to plan for the future, it is also important to focus on the present moment and enjoy the time you have with loved ones and pursuing your passions.

Remember, planning for the future with cancer can be overwhelming, and it is normal to experience a range of emotions. By working with your healthcare team, considering your priorities, making legal and financial arrangements, seeking support, and focusing on the present moment, you can make informed decisions about your care and find peace in the midst of uncertainty.

ADVANCED HEALTHCARE PLANNING WITH CANCER

Advance care planning is an important part of planning for the future with cancer. Advance care planning involves making decisions about your healthcare preferences in advance, so that your wishes can be respected if you are unable to make decisions for yourself.

Here are some things to consider when it comes to advance care planning and cancer:

Consider your values and preferences:
Think about what is most important to you when it comes to your healthcare. This can include things like quality of life, pain management, and spiritual or religious beliefs.

Choose a healthcare proxy:
Choose someone you trust to make healthcare decisions for you if you are unable to make them for yourself. Make sure to discuss your wishes with this person in advance.

Make a living will:
A living will is a legal document that outlines your healthcare preferences, including things like whether you would want to be resuscitated, receive artificial nutrition and hydration, or receive palliative care.

Communicate with your healthcare team:
Make sure that your healthcare team is aware of your advance care planning preferences. This can help to ensure that your wishes are respected if you are unable to communicate them yourself.

Review and update your plan regularly:
Your healthcare preferences may change over time, so it is important to review and update your plan regularly to ensure that it reflects your current wishes.

Advance care planning can help to ensure that your wishes are respected and that you receive care that is aligned with your values and preferences. By considering your values and preferences, choosing a healthcare proxy, making a living will, communicating with your healthcare team, and reviewing and updating your plan regularly, you can take an active role in planning for your future with cancer.

FINANCIAL PLANNING AND CANCER

Cancer treatment can be expensive, and it is important to consider financial planning as part of your overall plan for coping with cancer. Here are some tips for financial planning when facing cancer:

Understand your insurance coverage: Understand the details of your health insurance coverage, including copays, deductibles, and out-of-pocket maximums. Talk to your insurance provider or employer about any questions you have.

Ask about financial assistance programs:

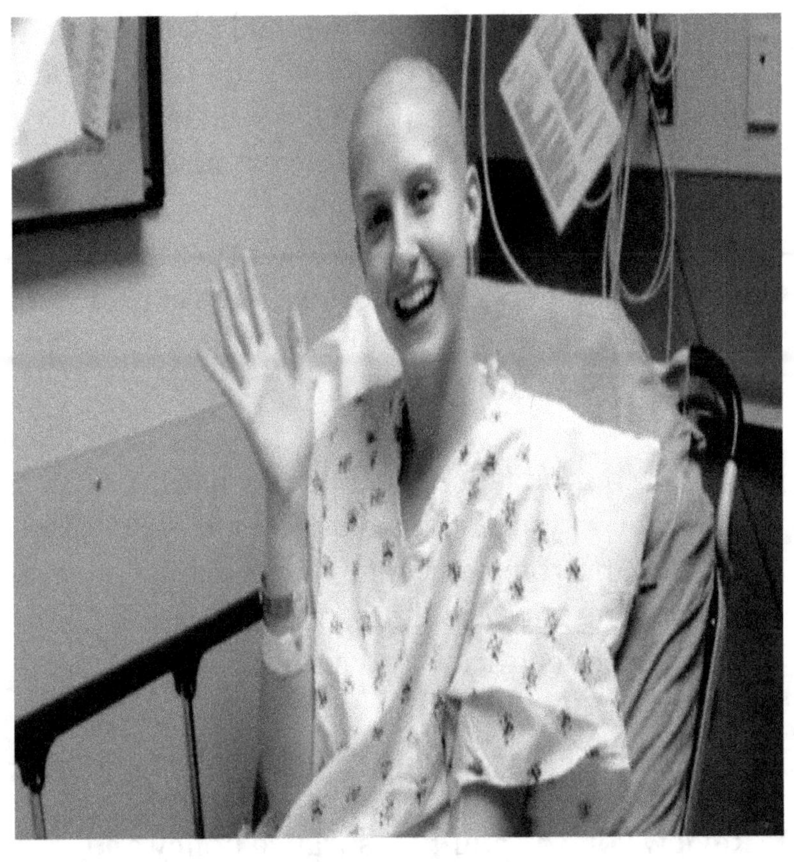

Many hospitals and cancer centers offer financial assistance programs for patients who are struggling to pay for treatment. These programs may include grants, financial counseling, and other resources.

Consider working with a financial planner: A financial planner can help you understand your financial situation and develop a plan to manage your expenses and investments.

Create a budget: Create a budget that includes your anticipated expenses related to cancer treatment, as well as other expenses such as rent, utilities, and groceries.

Explore options for reducing expenses: Consider ways to reduce your expenses, such as refinancing your mortgage or car loan, negotiating with creditors, or seeking out lower-cost healthcare providers.

Review your disability insurance and other benefits:
Review your disability insurance policy and other benefits to see if you are eligible for any financial assistance during your treatment.

Plan for the future:
Consider creating a financial plan that takes into account your long-term financial goals, such as retirement or college savings.

Remember, financial planning can be a complex
and emotional process. Don't hesitate to reach
out for help and support from a financial
planner, a social worker, or other professionals.
By taking an active role in financial planning,
you can help to minimize the financial impact
of cancer treatment and reduce stress on you
and your family.

Chapter Thirteen: END OF LIFE CHOICES AND CANCER

End-of-life planning is an important part of coping with cancer, and it can help to ensure that your wishes are respected and that your loved ones are supported. Here are some things to consider when it comes to end-of-life planning with cancer:

Choose a healthcare proxy:
Choose someone you trust to make healthcare decisions for you if you are unable to make them for yourself. Make sure to discuss your wishes with this person in advance.

Make a living will:
A living will is a legal document that outlines your healthcare preferences, including things like whether you would want to be resuscitated, receive artificial nutrition and hydration, or receive palliative care.

Consider palliative care:
Palliative care focuses on improving quality of life for patients with serious illnesses, and it can be an important part of end-of-life care. Talk to your healthcare team about whether palliative care may be appropriate for you.

Make funeral arrangements:
Consider making arrangements for your funeral or memorial service in advance. This can help to ensure that your wishes are respected and that your loved ones are not burdened with these decisions during a difficult time.

Discuss your wishes with loved ones:
 Talk to your loved ones about your wishes for end-of-life care and other important decisions. This can help to ensure that your wishes are respected and that your loved ones are prepared for what may come.

Remember, end-of-life planning can be a difficult and emotional process. Don't hesitate to seek out support from a counselor, social worker, or other professional. By taking an active role in end-of-life planning, you can help to ensure that your wishes are respected and that your loved ones are supported during a difficult time.

Chapter Fourteen: HEALTH TIPS TO PREVENT CANCER

There is no surefire way to prevent cancer, but there are several steps you can take to reduce your risk:

Eat a healthy diet:
A diet rich in fruits, vegetables, and whole grains can help to reduce your risk of cancer. Aim to eat a variety of colorful fruits and vegetables, and limit your intake of processed and red meats.

Maintain a healthy weight:
Being overweight or obese can increase your risk of several types of cancer. Aim to maintain a healthy weight through a balanced diet and regular exercise.

Exercise regularly:
Regular exercise can help to reduce your risk of several types of cancer. Aim for at least 150 minutes of moderate-intensity exercise per week, such as brisk walking or cycling.

Protect your skin:
Skin cancer is the most common type of cancer in the United States. Protect your skin from the sun by wearing protective clothing, using sunscreen with an SPF of 30 or higher, and avoiding tanning beds.

Quit smoking:
Smoking is the leading cause of preventable death in the United States and is responsible for several types of cancer. Quitting smoking can greatly reduce your risk of cancer.

Limit alcohol intake:
Alcohol consumption has been linked to several types of cancer, including breast, liver, and colon cancer. Limit your alcohol intake to no more than one drink per day for women and two drinks per day for men.

Get regular cancer screenings:
Regular cancer screenings can help to detect cancer early when it is most treatable. Talk to your healthcare provider about what screenings

are appropriate for you based on your age and other risk factors.

Limit exposure to radiation:
Exposure to ionizing radiation, such as from medical imaging tests or radiation therapy, can increase your risk of cancer. Talk to your healthcare provider about the risks and benefits of any imaging or treatment options, and consider limiting unnecessary exposure to radiation.

Avoid or limit processed foods:
Processed foods, such as packaged snacks and fast food, are often high in unhealthy fats, sugars, and additives, and may increase your risk of cancer. Try to eat whole foods as much as possible, and limit your intake of processed and packaged foods.

Eat a variety of healthy fats:
 Certain healthy fats, such as omega-3 fatty acids, may help to reduce your risk of cancer. Aim to include sources of healthy fats, such as fatty fish, nuts, and seeds, in your diet.

Get enough vitamin D:
Vitamin D has been linked to a reduced risk of several types of cancer. Try to get enough vitamin D through sunlight exposure, food sources (such as fatty fish and fortified dairy products), or supplements if recommended by your healthcare provider.

Practice safe sex:
Certain sexually transmitted infections, such as HPV, can increase your risk of cancer. Practice safe sex, including using condoms and getting vaccinated if appropriate.

Be aware of workplace hazards:
Exposure to certain workplace hazards, such as asbestos or diesel exhaust, can increase your risk of cancer. Be aware of potential hazards in your workplace, and take steps to limit your exposure where possible.

Stay socially connected:
Social isolation and loneliness have been linked to an increased risk of several types of cancer. Stay socially connected with friends and family,

and consider joining community groups or clubs to meet new people.

Remember, every individual's risk of cancer is different, and there is no one-size-fits-all approach to cancer prevention. Talk to your healthcare provider about what steps you can take to reduce your personal risk of cancer.

Chapter Fifteen: CONCLUSIVE ADVICE

Living with Cancer: Coping Strategies and Support

A cancer diagnosis can be a life-changing event that affects every aspect of your life. While it is normal to feel overwhelmed, scared, or uncertain about the future, there are many strategies and resources available to help you cope with the challenges of cancer and live as fully as possible.

Here are some tips and advice for living with cancer:

Build a Support System:
Reach out to family, friends, and healthcare professionals for emotional, practical, and medical support. Consider joining a cancer support group, where you can connect with others who are going through similar experiences.

Take Care of Your Physical Health:
Eat a healthy diet, get regular exercise, and take time to rest and relax. This can help improve your overall physical and emotional health, as well as reduce some of the side effects of cancer and its treatments.

Stay Informed:
 Learn as much as you can about your cancer diagnosis, treatment options, and supportive care services. This can help you make informed decisions and feel more in control of your cancer journey.

Focus on What You Can Control:
While cancer can feel overwhelming and out of your control, focus on the things that you can control, such as your daily routines, self-care practices, and treatment decisions.

Manage Stress:
Chronic stress can weaken the immune system and increase inflammation in the body, which can contribute to cancer risk. Practice

stress-reducing techniques such as meditation, deep breathing, or yoga.

Communicate Effectively:
Effective communication with your healthcare team and loved ones can help you get the support and care that you need. Be open and honest about your feelings, concerns, and needs.

Take Advantage of Supportive Care Services:
Supportive care services, such as pain management, palliative care, and hospice care, can help improve your quality of life and manage symptoms related to cancer and its treatments.

Remember, every individual's cancer journey is unique, and there is no one-size-fits-all approach to living with cancer. Take the time to find what works best for you, and don't be afraid to ask for help when you need it. With the right support and care, it is possible to live a fulfilling life with cancer.